South Asian disabled young people and their families

Yasmin Hussain, Karl Atkin and Waqar Ahmad

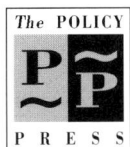

The POLICY
P~P
PRESS

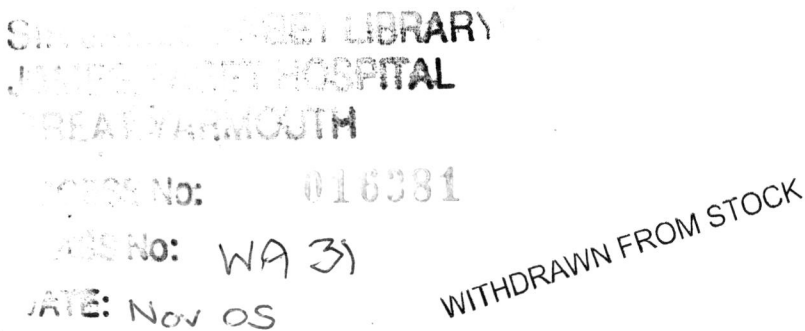
First published in Great Britain in July 2002 by

The Policy Press
34 Tyndall's Park Road
Bristol BS8 1PY
UK

Tel no +44 (0)117 954 6800
Fax no +44 (0)117 973 7308
E-mail tpp@bristol.ac.uk
www.policypress.org.uk

Published for the Joseph Rowntree Foundation by The Policy Press

ISBN 1 86134 326 4

Yasmin Hussain is Research Fellow, Department of Social Policy and Sociology, **Karl Atkin** is Senior Lecturer, Centre for Research in Primary Care and **Waqar Ahmad** was Professor of Primary Care Research and Director of the Centre for Research in Primary Care during the project, all at the University of Leeds.

The **Joseph Rowntree Foundation** has supported this project as part of its programme of research and innovative development projects, which it hopes will be of value to policy makers, practitioners and service users. The facts presented and views expressed in this report are, however, those of the authors and not necessarily those of the Foundation.

The statements and opinions contained within this publication are solely those of the authors and contributors and not of The University of Bristol or The Policy Press. The University of Bristol and The Policy Press disclaim responsibility for any injury to persons or property resulting from any material published in this publication.

The Policy Press works to counter discrimination on grounds of gender, race, disability, age and sexuality.

Front cover: image of tree blossom supplied by DigitalVision
Cover design by Qube Design Associates, Bristol
Printed in Great Britain by Hobbs the Printers Ltd, Southampton

Contents

Acknowledgements

Our greatest debt is to the young people, their parents, brothers and sisters who shared their experience with us. Considerable thanks must also go to the many professionals who gave freely of their time and goodwill in helping the project. Particular thanks go to Zoebia Ali, Ghazanfar Bhatti, Paul Bywaters, Elaine Evans, Khalid Hussain, Saeed Lunat, Alyas Karmani, Anita Pierides and Mike Smith.

Hazel Blackburn provided invaluable administrative and secretarial support. We are also grateful to our many colleagues at the Centre for Research in Primary Care, who were supportive of our work and willing to listen and offer advice. Special thanks go to Lesley Jones and Angela Hemingway, who helped edit this report.

The Joseph Rowntree Foundation provided financial support for the project. Emma Stone, our liaison officer, provided helpful guidance and support.

Finally, we benefited from the expertise of the advisory committee: Bryony Beresford, Suleman Chunara, Aliya Darr, Asif Hussain, Alison O'Sullivan, Mark Priestley, Mohammed Shabir, Iain Smith, Emma Stone, Selina Ullah and Ayesha Vernon. Our thanks to all these people, whose support was vital to the successful completion of the project.

Introduction

Aims of the research

This report is about the views of South Asian young people with impairments. We wanted to find out how everyday lives were reflected in policy and practice. Little is known about young people from minority ethnic communities with impairments and this sometimes affects how they are treated by the services. Myths and stereotypes about different ethnic groups can lead to discrimination. Policy and practice are not always based on what people actually want. This study set out to understand the views young people and their families had about their lives in order to try to improve this situation.

We aimed to find out about:

- ideas about impairment and disability among young South Asian people;
- what they and their families thought of the formal and informal support which they received;
- how gender, age and friendships affect the experience of impairment;
- how much the experience of white people with impairments might influence services used by South Asian people;
- the effects of culture, religion and ethnicity on young people's lives.

We started from the everyday experience of the young people themselves. We talked to young people about their families, friends and networks as well as the changes they were making in their lives such as school and work and how they saw the future. We looked at what had been written before about these topics by other people and some of our own work on disability and chronic illness, with regard to people from minority ethnic communities.

The research methods

The project was carried out by Yasmin Hussain, Karl Atkin and Waqar Ahmad from the Centre for Research in Primary Care, University of Leeds.

We spoke to 29 disabled young people: 16 young men and 13 young women. We were keen to see how disabled and non-disabled people got through times of change (education, work, possibly living away from home, building their own families). We included people who were aged between 17- and 30-years-old. (See the Appendix for more details about the people we interviewed.)

Nineteen young people were Muslim and 10 were Sikh. We could not find anyone Hindu to interview although we tried very hard to do so. This was partly because of the area in which we were working but also reflected difficulties which we had experienced before in other work. One Hindu brother was interviewed but unfortunately we could not interview the young person with the impairment. All the respondents had left school.

We also talked to 14 parents (eight described themselves as Muslim, six as Sikh) and 15 brothers and sisters. We contacted them through the young people themselves. We interviewed brothers and sisters, so we could compare the disabled young person's experience with someone of a similar age and gender in the family.

We were introduced to young people by various organisations (both statutory and voluntary) from West Yorkshire and a small number from the West Midlands, as well as by community members. This was especially important because we wanted to include young people who might not be in touch with services. The interviews with young people were mostly done at home, although seven wanted to meet somewhere else. Parents were interviewed at home.

We wanted to ask about what they thought of disability and the barriers, attitudes and discrimination they experienced rather than the medical effects of impairment. Some young people included in the study had been born with impairments, others experienced impairments later on, including cerebral palsy, multiple sclerosis, arthritis and impairments because of strokes and accidental injury.

The young people and their families were offered a choice of interviewer (male or female) and which language they wanted to be interviewed in. Ten interviews were in Punjabi, one in Urdu, and 47 were in English.

We used qualitative research methods because we were interested in what young South Asian people and their families thought of their lives from their different perspectives. We also wanted to know about the other influences on them, how they saw impairment, religion, ethnicity, culture, age and gender and what they thought of themselves and how others saw them as well as their experience of different types of discrimination.

We wanted to find out about the way that disability worked to stop people doing the things that they wanted to do and how much they felt left out or looked down upon because of it. Having an impairment is made worse if you feel that people treat you badly – is that discrimination different for South Asian young people and does it affect the way the services work?

We were interested in young people's lives. This report was carried out against a background of policy initiatives such as Quality Protects, reports such as *Excellence not excuses: A jigsaw of services* (SSI, 2000) and *They look after their own don't they?* (SSI, 1998), and legislation such as the 2000 Race Relations Amendment Act. Changes are taking place which may be having an impact on policy and practice in relation to institutional racism.

Young people's views on identity: religion, culture and ethnicity

This chapter is about how young people see themselves, and the influences of religion, culture and ethnicity.

A positive perspective on disability can help give young people a strong view of themselves. The social model of disability, though, can also reflect a Eurocentric view, that of white culture, which might seem to undermine other cultural, religious and ethnic values. Independence and autonomy, for example, may be interpreted differently and they might not have the same meaning among different ethnic groups. Bignall and Butt (2000) found this to be true in their study of black disabled young people.

For young South Asian people in the UK, ideas of independence might be a combination of their parents' ethnic, cultural and religious values as well as those of the broader British culture. This is why independence might be as important to South Asian young people living in the UK as to their white counterparts, but it may be expressed quite differently. The accounts of young people and their parents reflect this. Robina's mother said:

"But I think within our culture it's difficult ... like I couldn't say to my parents like I'm going to live independently, like an English person could do that, there would be difficulties."

This is not to say that the parents and young people had no sense of independence. Indeed, many mentioned it as important. Young people were especially irritated if their parents tried to restrict their attempts to become independent. Developing some separation from their parents and having some control over their own lives,

however, was not always associated with leaving home and living away. The young people tried to balance having more control over their lives with being dependent on one another within the family – and giving and taking. More generally, being independent was a part of young people's desire to value their ethnic, cultural and religious differences. It became important both in their experience of disability and in its own right, as an important part of identity. This seems to be the case for the 'second generation', whether or not they have an impairment. Academic, policy and everyday discussions tend to put a lot of emphasis on 'cultural conflict' between young people and their parents. Literature on relations between generations, however, describes social change but also culture being passed down to the next generation. Does impairment or disability change that and is it influenced by ethnic, religious and cultural factors?

Ethnicity

It is not easy to define ethnicity. The term includes language, culture, religion, nationality and a shared history. It is also seen as a political symbol which marks out being excluded by a powerful majority but also solidarity with others in similar situations. It was significant to ask young people and their families their views on the subject.

Contact with the country where their parents came from could be a large part of identity and such links were important for nearly all the parents. Impairment did have an effect on these links. Several young people and their families were reluctant to visit their countries of origin because of the practical difficulties of air travel and organising the trip. Young people and their parents also felt that the support available in the UK would not be so readily available in Pakistan or India. Some of the other reasons families gave for not visiting their homeland were about the way South Asian societies saw impairment and disability. Both young people and their parents felt that, despite the negative view of disability in the UK, disability carried a greater sense of stigma and discrimination in South Asian countries.

Young people with impairments and their brothers and sisters had a mixed view of their parents' homeland, as do many other South Asian young people living in the UK. Gurubax's brother has never been to India and does not feel any particular links to his parents' homeland: "I come from here". Gurubax shared this view. More young people and their brothers and sisters identified with being 'British' than being 'Pakistani' or 'Indian'. Their sense of Britishness was often matter of fact because of being born and living in Britain. Mushtaq's brother said, "England's my country really, just here, I'm used to here and everything". Young people and their brothers and sisters also had a strong sense of being British because they compared what was available to them in the UK and in South Asia. As part of this, there was a general sense that the views held by the South Asian community living in the UK were less rigid than those of their parents' homeland. Waseem's sister disliked Pakistan: "It's very narrow minded". Some of the young people with impairment often described themselves as British, and linked this to disability and being given more 'respect' in Britain than Pakistan or India. The negative experiences mentioned before perhaps added to the young people's sense of being British; Britain was associated with being more 'disabled-friendly'. So having a disability could influence the young person's view of where they belonged.

Their parents valued trips to their homeland. However, they thought that children learning their community language was more important than keeping in touch with the parental homeland. Young people and their sisters and brothers shared this view and this explained why many of them could speak a language other than English. Both Fatima and her sister had learnt Punjabi. Her sister said, "otherwise it's like losing your own language". However, several disabled young people had not been encouraged to learn their

parents' language, unlike their brothers and sisters. Sometimes this was seen as part of disability, for instance, if they had speech impairments. In other cases it was because the family felt the young person had enough to cope with, besides learning another language. Again the effect of impairment should not be made too much of. Some of the brothers and sisters we interviewed could not speak their parents' language either. How much the parents emphasised their ties with their homeland and the learning of their language was the key to the responses of their children. If the parents had little interest, for example, it was unlikely that any of their children had strong ties with their parents' country of birth or whether they spoke their parents' language.

Religion and culture

Religion also offered an identity for a South Asian young person living in the UK and one that was assumed to be very important for families. Gurucharan's mother said that all her children were keen to learn about religion:

> "It is important. If you don't take them to the temple then they do not know about religion. We are not like white people and we make sure our children know about religion."

Muslim parents said the same sort of things and religious observance was usually valued. Nargis' father wanted all his children to learn about their religion and go to the mosque: "It gives you peace of mind, a sense of self-worth and it tells you who you are". Parents felt sad if they saw impairment interfering with their child's religious education.

In fact, several young people did not have the same access to religion and culture as their non-impaired brothers and sisters. Nineteen-year-old Tahir did not know much about religion and he contrasted his knowledge with that of his brothers who were able to read the Qur'an and attend the mosque: "I don't go to the mosque because I'm disabled and they don't teach me nothing". Significantly, some of the parents – all Muslim – felt their child's impairment excused them from religious practices. Tahir's mother described how her son's impairment meant that he did not learn the Qur'an: "It would be too much to ask". Her other children, however, did learn about Islam. Isma's mother took a similar view, feeling that her daughter was unable to practise religion: "Allah understands this. Islam gives priority for the disabled". Twenty-four-year-old Mushtaq's brother said his brother knew nothing about religion:

> "I don't think he even knows how to read [the Qur'an]. I don't know. Because I don't think my mum's ever taught him. I think my mum thought he was disabled and you know he doesn't really need to know that much."

Even among the majority of families who wanted their children to learn about religion, young people experienced difficulties. They often had poor access to wider community networks. Many felt isolated within their own South Asian communities and this did not help them to practise their religion. A particular problem was religious education. There was an emphasis on rote learning in both mosques and temples and on using other spoken languages for religious instruction (usually Urdu, Punjabi or Hindi). Teachers sometimes failed to accommodate the young person's impairment or did little to support or encourage them. Inzimam knew less about religious teaching than his non-disabled brothers. He was made to feel different when he attended the mosque and was taught in a separate room, away from the other children. Furthermore, he added, "the Imam did not seem that interested in teaching him". Moeen's mother said that the Imam had told her son, who had an impairment, to stay at home, yet he was willing to teach her other children. The young people themselves were also unhappy with the reception they got when they attended religious services. Azhar was disappointed that his brothers and sisters knew more about religion than he did. He felt that this was because he did not feel welcome in the mosque on account of his cerebral palsy. So Azhar no longer went there. Hardeep had stopped going to the temple because of people staring at her. Gurudev's mother used to go to the temple with her son but did not go anymore because of the lack of disabled access. There may be limited resources for mosques' and temples' religious instruction classes but the fact remains that disabled young people found them unsupportive places. Religious communities need to address the disabling barriers which they create

by isolating or discriminating against people with impairments.

Some of the Sikh families came across theological barriers to learning about religion as well as practical ones. For some of these families their child's impairment was associated with the sins of a previous life. This view reflected the response of the wider Sikh community, even if the parent did not agree with it. Jagjeet's mother explained that other people in the Sikh community believed that she was being punished for past life sins:

> "It's like the olders (sic), you know, they assume that I've been punished for something that I must have done, something wrong in my past life."

It is not surprising that most of the Sikh young people themselves did not usually believe this account of disability; it would have been potentially damaging to their idea of themselves. Sometimes tensions occurred in the family because of it. Gurupal remarked that his mother felt his impairment was because of sins in a past life:

> "I think my mum found it very difficult to accept the fact that I was disabled when I was born, because she thought it was a sort of punishment from God, like she had done something bad and that's why she had a disabled son."

He, however, did not agree with this:

> "Look, I am what I am and God has made me the way I am and there's nothing I can do to change that, so we just accept me for myself and don't sort of like bringing religion into it because religion has got nothing to do with it."

Muslims usually took a more positive view. Impairment was seen as given by Allah, who would also provide the resources to cope with it. This idea was not very often accepted completely. A few Muslim families expressed anger with God for 'giving them' a child with an impairment. Similar views were expressed by some Sikh families, although being angry in the long term was the exception rather than the rule.

The lack of religious knowledge among the disabled young people with impairments seemed to be largely about the more formal rituals, such as reading the Qur'an and praying. This put them at a disadvantage compared to their brothers and sisters. Twenty-eight-year-old Fatima, like some of the other young people, described how impairment interfered with her ability to practise religion:

"Well I can't read the Namas [prayers], like properly, like standing up because I can't sit down on the floor, I find it difficult."

Actually, no young person was completely removed from their parents' religion, culture and ethnicity. Some said that impairment had not interfered with their religious education at all. Thirty-year-old Gurubax said he had learned about religion in the same way as his brothers; there had been no difference between them in his view. Several young people said that practising religion was so important that disability would not create any barriers. Those who drew strength from religion held this view. Inzimam went to the mosque when he was upset:

"I normally go to the mosque or read the Qur'an or something like that, you know, which I usually do; my disability doesn't come into it."

Most of the young people we interviewed had a good working knowledge of religion and culture and were a part of their family's religious and cultural lives. Although twenty-year-old Robina no longer went to the mosque because she resented people staring at her – adult women's attendance at a mosque is generally less common compared to men's – she still felt that religion was important to her:

"It's just you've been born into the religion, that's where your family background lies, so yes it is important to me.

Robina was able to learn about Islam by reading at home and talking with her family. Most young people knew enough about their family's religion and culture to feel that they did belong to their religious community as well as knowing how to behave 'appropriately'.

Social change

Learning about one type of culture or religion while living in another (sometimes hostile) culture is a difficulty faced by people from minority ethnic groups. Young people may be open to influences which many parents would wish to protect them from. This account by nineteen-year-old Nargis' father was typical:

"I would rather they stick to our traditional culture. I would rather have my daughters wear traditional dress because of our culture."

Young people with an impairment and their brothers and sisters usually respected these attitudes, although they began to question some of their parents' values, as they adopted more Western ones. This rarely led to direct conflict as these other Western values were considered alongside – and not instead of – their parents' values. What is of particular interest is that both the young person and the rest of the family saw change in similar ways. Working out change involving religion, culture and ethnicity needs a lot of understanding as well as social skills. Impairment could affect this, but not fundamentally, and young people did seem to have enough understanding to accommodate these various influences on their lives, without being too confrontational. So the young people with impairments were not particularly disadvantaged in this respect and had various ways of avoiding conflict with their parents. This was usually done through interpreting cultural rules and avoiding open displays of offensive behaviour: this might be seen as something common to keeping relationships going generally.

Conflicts that did arise between parents and young people were as much about understanding cultural values as a lack of knowledge of these values. Some young people, for example, challenged their parents' restrictions about clothes by arguing that these were based on 'ethnic culture' rather than on 'religious values'. These distinctions were seen as important and were used to argue for relaxation of restrictions. Young people and their brothers and sisters also had a strong interest in youth culture, but again often within the framework of their families, religion and culture. Modesty, for example, was valued by many of the young women – irrespective of impairment – and offered another example of how well the parents had passed on their culture. Fatima (aged 28) knew that she should be modest, but said this could be done with both 'traditional' and western clothes. Her parents were happy with this and Fatima successfully responded to their worries:

"No, I mean my mum and dad, they prefer if we wore traditional clothes at home, but if we're going out to work, or going to college or university, they've never stopped us wearing trousers. But that doesn't mean we'd go and wear short skirts, things, you know show our legs, sort of things. As long as we're covered, they don't mind. Otherwise, I think they would get too upset, my family."

Twenty-eight-year-old Gurupal said that his parents did not understand him, but added that they did not understand his brothers and sisters either. He put this down to cultural differences between young people and parents. The parents, he said, still held on to the 'old ways of doing things'. This caused tensions, but Gurupal had enough skills to negotiate these tensions. He was aware that his older brother had to go through the same things with his parents, but pointed out that becoming independent was particularly difficult for himself. His parents did not like him going to clubs and public houses, for example. First, because they felt that it was culturally wrong and second because they worried that his impairment made him at risk. Gurupal said:

"I really had to stamp my foot down and say, 'Mum, I respect your opinion and I appreciate what you're saying and I'm taking this on board', but I mean I can't be stuck in the house for all of my life and staring at four walls, I have to socialise and interact with people, because that is the only way I'm going to develop as a person."

Gurupal's experience showed how young people had to engage with both the effects of disabling ideas about them as well as cultural expectations when negotiating with their parents.

Gender and culture

Ideas about how men and women should behave played an important part in how parents saw their children's friendships. They worried about the effect of damage to their daughter's reputation, for instance. Young women were seen by parents as needing greater protection than men. Gender seemed more important than impairment in parents' attempts to protect their children. Jagjeet's mother summed up the concerns of many of them: "Sons are sons, they're boys. You don't worry about boys, do you, the same way?" The young women, themselves, recognised these differences too.

Most respected their parents' views but some young women – irrespective of impairment – were beginning to voice criticisms and commented on the unfairness of such different treatment. Twenty-eight-year-old Fatima said her parents kept a closer eye on her because she was a woman. Her brother with an impairment had more freedom:

"My brother's got no pressure at all, I mean he comes in and out, it's like you don't even know where he is, he could be anywhere. Whereas I go away for a minute and they want to know where you are."

She added that "in Asian families there was no such thing as equal opportunities" with regard to gender. Waseem's sister agreed and said that her family treated her differently to her brother:

"There is no problem if my brothers have girlfriends. And I was like, 'how come it's alright for him to go out with someone, when he's a male, when it's not fine for me to find someone out there'. I said, 'Mum, you're spoken like a typical Asian now and I thought you didn't have a backward view'.... Since I've turned 16, it's like most of their attention has gone on me, more protective of me and I think maybe, I don't know, something that Asian families go through, you know, when their daughters gets to that age."

Impairment did influence the families' ideas about young men's and women's relationships. Young disabled men were given more concessions, sometimes almost as compensation for impairment. Threats to the reputations of their daughters with impairments, however, were dealt with by restrictions on their access to the outside world. Female reputations were seen as more easily damaged and less easy to repair than male reputations within South Asian communities. Nineteen-year-old Nargis' father did not like his daughter attending social clubs with other disabled people: "I don't want her to go along with [the idea] that girls should have male friends". Young women with impairments tended to be more isolated than young men in the same situation.

Summary

This chapter explored how young people saw ethnicity, religion and culture:

- Although impairment affected their religious and cultural knowledge, it did not seem as important as the value placed on these things by the rest of the family. On the whole, if parents stressed the importance of religion, so did the young people and their brothers and sisters.
- Generally, the chapter shows how impairment is only one part of a young person's identity. Other social factors, including culture and religion, being male or female and the experience of racial discrimination influenced how they experienced disability and impairment.
- Young people felt that their parents were more protective of their daughters than their sons and worried more about their daughters' reputations.

Views on marriage and family

3

"You know what grannies are like, always nagging."

This section is about views the people we interviewed had on marriage and the family. It includes family obligations and how ideas about disability and impairment are worked out within the family.

Part of the family

Some parents saw impairment as a tragedy that made their child more at risk than others. Parents, for example, could be 'overprotective', often underestimating their sons' and daughters' abilities as well as the amount of control they had over their lives. In fact, parents often felt responsible for all aspects of their child's life. They concentrated on markers which they saw as 'normal' for their children: a good education; social skills; knowledge of their religion and culture; as well as having a job and getting married. Parents worried about all their children but were more concerned for their son or daughter with an impairment because they saw them as needing extra looking after. They also were aware of the changing nature of the problems faced by young people as they got older. Parents expected to be involved in the life of their son or daughter who had an impairment far longer than they did for their other children. Such ideas sometimes set up tensions between the young people and their parents. Nineteen-year-old Moeen's mother summed up the views of many parents:

"I want him to go out, but ... I worry about him. I always think that something might happen to him."

A particular worry mentioned by nearly all the mothers and fathers was what would happen to their son or daughter after their own deaths. Clearly this is a common worry among parents of a son or daughter with a chronic illness or disability – of all ethnic groups. The parents whom we interviewed, however, did not worry about their other children in the same way, it seemed, since they felt they would find it easier to get support, find a job and be financially independent. Parents were concerned that their child with an impairment would not have the same opportunities as the other children. Nagina's mother felt extreme concern when thinking about her daughter's future:

"Sometimes I pray, 'before I go, God, take her first' because I don't want to leave her behind me. I have six daughters, but when they get married, they have their own life, you know, they have their children, their husband, another life."

These comments also reflect the different attitudes to young men and women. Young South Asian women, once married, may have few responsibilities towards their family of birth. Instead, they are regarded as members of their husband's household. Having sons, however, did not always reassure the parent that their child with an impairment would be looked after in the future. Thirty-year-old Gurudev's mother did not expect his brothers or sisters to look after him:

"Nowadays everyone is so busy with their own lives, they've got no time for anybody, have they?"

Several other parents were concerned about changes in the family obligations and contrasted unfavourably the present generations' 'more Western' expectations with those of their own generations. Rabia's father explained:

"Here children do not look after their parents, let alone their sisters, do they? Don't get me wrong, all her brothers and sisters, all would give their life for her, they love her even more than us. But it's not the same as it used to be. Those from Pakistan would look after people like Rabia. People born here are very reluctant to do that."

Many parents expressed similar views. Some were especially pessimistic because their other sons and daughters offered little current support. This did not, they felt, bode well for the future. Moeen's mother was disappointed about the role of her other sons:

"Nowadays children won't do what they are told; they do what they want. Other children help their parents, but they [her sons] don't do anything."

Not all parents, however, shared these anxieties. Many hoped their other children would continue to be involved in the care of their son or daughter with an impairment. What did those brothers and sisters think? Twenty-six-year-old Hardeep's brother was one of the few we interviewed who felt that his sister was not his responsibility. Most had a more ambivalent response. They were, for example, aware of the difficulties of supporting their brothers or sisters themselves after they have left the family home to get married. Shushma's sister said that she would be married soon and was worried about who would then look after her sister when she left home. At present she was responsible for the daily care of her sister. Nonetheless, thirty-year-old Gurucharan's brother felt that he would always have a duty to support Gurucharan:

"It's been tough on us actually. It's a lot of headache for us. We're always there for him and we've always wanted to be there for him.... We're a close-knit family in the sense that we're always there. I know that he'd

do the same for me, if I were in that situation, so I couldn't really turn away. These sorts of things, misfortunate things can happen to anyone."

For many brothers and sisters, this was seen as continuation of the support they already gave. Like their parents, they felt that they had an obligation to support all their family. Twenty-eight-year-old Fatima's sister remarked, "My mum does everything during the day, so we've got to come home and at least help out". Again, being a young woman was an important influence on this sense of obligation. Sisters were expected to help out more within the family than brothers. Fatima's sister, for example, felt she was put under more pressure by her family to look after Fatima than her brothers were.

Worrying about the future of their sons and daughters who had impairments meant many parents hoped that they could find a suitable marriage partner to 'look after' their child, although they felt that this would be far from straightforward. Another strategy adopted by several parents was to encourage the young person towards greater independence. Nineteen-year-old Tahir's mother said:

"I try to make him independent. I think that is where a lot of mothers went wrong and they give the child everything. If they don't give the child everything, they've got to go and get it and that encourages the child to get up and go."

Many parents had to struggle with their own negative views of disability and this sometimes worked against the idea of independence for their child. It was common, for example, for many families to say that they tried to treat all their children in the same way. Thirty-year-old Gurupal's mother remarked:

"We have never treated him differently. We just treat him as normal, we never think of him as disabled, well yeah he is disabled to look at but we are there to help him. I don't know, we always treat him the same as others."

Both young people and their brothers' and sisters' accounts largely confirmed this approach. Parents realised that it did not always work, because they felt that they could not fully avoid the implications of their son's or daughter's impairment. Several parents were aware, for instance, that they sometimes spent more time with the young person with an impairment than with their other children. This often caused problems. Nineteen-year-old Tahir's mother remarked that in the past she focused too much on her eldest son at the expense of his younger brothers and sisters:

> "We wrapped him so much in cotton wool, we forgot about the other children and the other kids were left out and it's not fair. They started arguing between themselves. There was jealousy."

Brothers and sisters noticed this too and often felt the brother or sister with the impairment was given preferential treatment. According to 19-year-old Nargis' brother:

> "I felt left out all the time, because everybody cares for her more than me. Especially my dad, he always says Nargis comes first."

Most accepted this, although they admitted there were times when they were resentful. They were also aware of how their brother's or sister's impairment had had an impact on their own lives and the opportunities which were available to them. Twenty-eight-year-old Fatima's sister, for example, sometimes felt angry when she thought about how her sister's impairment has affected the family. This sister particularly wanted to leave home and go to university; the family were against this idea because they felt that she should stay at home and look after Fatima. The sister, however, kept her feelings about this hidden and even felt guilty about having such thoughts at all. Twenty-three-year-old Gurudyal's sister said she tried to support her brother and be positive, but admitted that there were occasions when she resented the time his parents give to her brother. Some brothers and sisters felt neglected. Jealousy was also a problem sometimes, as it is in most families, with or without family members with impairment.

Impairment and relationships

The parents' response to their child's impairment was not necessarily related to their ethnic background. South Asian families seem to subscribe to the same negative views of impairment held by white families. There were loving relationships between young people and their families, however, despite these views. This was true of both those still living at home and those who lived away. Nasira praised her family:

> "They help me a lot. And you know, they'll do a lot for me. My family supports me 100%. They make life easier for me. And I've got a family; I don't really need anybody else, do I? They care for me really a lot."

The families also emphasised their love for the young person. Tahir's mother was very close to her son:

> "If anything happens to him now, I don't know what I would do. I don't. I would be really lost. I really would be lost."

Families and young people worked at getting on well together and nearly all described a supportive family atmosphere. As a result, some families felt that their child's impairment had actually brought them closer together.

Such loving relationships were usually reflected in the families' attitude to looking after their relative. Parents of young people expressed a sense of love, but also of responsibility and moral obligation. Tahir's mother said:

> "I've been coping for six years. It's difficult to go through. Don't ask me where I've got the strength, I don't know. I just hope I've got the strength to carry on. Sometimes I've felt like, forget him, run away, but you can't, you cannot run away from it. It is impossible. They are your children and you have to look after them."

As in other relationships, everyday care usually fell to the mother, with the fathers undertaking other responsibilities. These good relationships did not, however, diminish the impact of support on the parents' life. Nineteen-year-old Nargis' father described how having a child with an impairment affected family life:

> "We're not allowed to get on with what we want to do. But we try and give her as much as we can."

Nagina's mother described a good relationship with her 'special' daughter but still felt that there were times when she found the pressure of caring was too much. Other parents shared this view. Caring had a big impact on parents' own (especially the mothers') lives. At times, they found caring physically hard, emotionally difficult and restricting their own social life and chances to work outside the home. These South Asian parents faced similar difficulties in providing practical, social and financial support to any other families in the same situation.

The young people with impairments, as well as their brothers and sisters, recognised the pressures faced by their parents. The young people in particular were aware of how much their parents had to go through and recognised that their mother and father sometimes had a sense of sadness and disappointment at having a child with an impairment. This seemed to emphasise a negative view of disability. Some young people expressed a sense of guilt for making life so difficult for their parents. Nineteen-year-old Nargis said it 'is not right' that her parents still have to look after her. Moeen was aware of tensions between his mother and father and believes that the pressures of looking after him directly contribute to their arguments. Twenty-two-year-old Jamila was aware of how upset her mother became and this worried her:

> "It's hard for mum to open up because she really gets upset and like she'll have tears in her eyes. It's really hard for her. But the thing is she's more upset than I am. I'm used to it."

Parents, however, remained vital allies for their children, offering encouragement and support. This meant there was a constant tension in their stories – similar to those described by their sons and daughters. As they tried to make sense of their own sadness at having a son or daughter with an impairment, they also wanted to make the most of the opportunities available to that young person and to have faith in their futures. Working out these tensions explains why some of the families' responses to disability did shift and change, at some times appearing contradictory. It explains, for instance, why some parents' ways of overcoming the disadvantages faced by their son or daughter might not always have been in the young person's best interests (despite their best intentions). Most parents attempted to adjust to

impairment by treating the children 'as if they were normal'. Such pressure to be normal sometimes ignores the reality of the impairment. This may also have benefits though. Indeed many young people said that this approach helped them to feel good about themselves. However, it did mean that parents sometimes failed to recognise the value of their children meeting other people with impairments or joining disabled groups.

The extended family

A stereotype which was challenged by the project's findings was that of the necessarily supportive extended South Asian family. Parents often criticised their extended family for having negative ideas about disability (despite these being similar to their own on some occasions). The extended family was seen as creating barriers for all of them. Young people and their sisters and brothers shared this opinion. These views within South Asian communities are perhaps no different from those of the general population. The study presented a picture of the extended family as a mixed blessing, sometimes oppressive, like a moral police force but providing little practical support. Shehnaz commented on another disadvantage of having relatives living close by: "A nightmare, I don't like it. It's too close, too close for comfort". Problems with the extended family were obviously not just a consequence of the child's impairment. Nargis and her sister's account of their relationship with their grandmother could be taken from any study on family relationships. Nineteen-year-old Nargis commented:

> "Grandma tells dad what to do. I really get mad at that. I don't know if she does it unintentionally, but it's not right. She gets on my nerves sometimes. You know what grannies are like, always nagging."

The extended family, however, could be a great help and some families spoke highly of such contact, praising the material, social and emotional help that they received. This support, however, was often greater in the early days of the impairment. Some families remarked that such support rarely continued and several parents felt that they had been left alone to look after their child. This general lack of support created tensions and led several families to contrast the unfavourable response of the extended family in the UK with the (perhaps mythical) attitudes in their homeland. Isma's father said:

"In Pakistan, they all think that our relatives in this country help us a lot, but they don't. When any family is in hard times, nobody wants to know at all."

The extended family could have other disadvantages. Those we talked to mentioned how their families often discriminated against them and how they found themselves socially isolated and left out of things. Families with a child with an impairment, for example, were not always welcome at family gatherings. Sushma's sister described a recent visit to her aunt's house:

"Everyone else is scared that she might break something and so will anticipate the worse and she went to my aunt's house the other day and everyone like said, 'why did you bring her, why did you bring her?'."

When families did attend such social events they often had to face negative comments. Young people with impairments, their parents and sisters and brothers wished that the extended families were more accommodating and understanding. Their lack of understanding caused sadness, anger and resentment.

Finding a marriage partner

Finding a job, or marrying or setting up home were seen as important symbols of growing up. Finding a suitable marriage partner can be a worry for parents and young people – with or without impairment. Parents did comment on how much more difficult it would be to find a marriage partner for their disabled child, compared to their other children. Both young people and their parents emphasised the importance of finding a partner who could offer support and care, but the difficulties in realising this were often a source of great sadness. Several young people were pessimistic. Twenty-seven-year-old Waheed wanted a wife but worried that he would end up alone:

"Obviously when my younger sister gets married, obviously she'll have to leave and my parents, my father is already 63 and my

mum is 50 something and when they pass away, I'll be on my own and I hate to be alone. And that really does choke me sometimes."

He added that his father was reluctant to approach other family members and ask about potential marriage partners:

"He thinks they will say, 'You know your son is disabled' and you know he's scared they might, you know, make fun of him and say 'why do this?' You know, 'Your son is disabled, are you stupid or what?' But deep down, he knows that they'll definitely refuse, so he goes, why bother to ask, you know."

Nineteen-year-old Nargis' father echoed this by saying that it will take time to find his daughter a marriage partner: "If she was normal, she would be married by now". Nineteen-year-old Shakeel shared similar feelings and remarked that he will never be able to get married:

"It falls into the category of things I cannot do. Because I'm too ill, that's why, even if there was someone who wanted to marry me. I wouldn't be able to get married to them because I wouldn't be able to look after them, they would probably have to end up looking after me."

Shakeel added that he tried not to dwell on this, as the thought of being alone depressed him:

"Well you do think about them things, but then if I think about them, I get depressed you see, so I try not to think about them."

Altogether, 11 of the young people we talked to were or had been married (including two who were now divorced). The experiences of those who had been married reflected the concerns of the unmarried young people and their parents. Thirty-year-old Gurudev said that his recent divorce was because his wife could not come to terms with his impairment, caused by a brain haemorrhage. Five other young people said they were on the verge of separation. Both Waseem (aged 27) and Gurucharan (aged 30) felt they were a 'burden' on their wives and unable to support their families in the way in which they felt that they should. To this extent, they saw impairment as a barrier to doing something that they had expected to – to have a successful married life. Impairment did not always have such a direct impact on relationships, however. Twenty-seven-year-old Hardeep rushed into marriage because she was worried that no one would want to marry her. She then regretted it, as she did not get on with her husband. There was no doubt, she said, that her impairment made her relationship with her husband more difficult, but she went on to say that that was not the 'real reason' for tensions in their relationship. It was simply that they shared different views on life and so were constantly arguing. Similarly, 30-year-old Jaswant said that she divorced her husband, not because of her multiple sclerosis, but because her husband had a 'controlling' personality and often bullied her. The experience of Jaswant and Hardeep showed that although impairment had an effect on young people's relationships, it was not the only cause of tensions and that these young people experienced similar relationship problems to all young people.

Despite some concerns, marriage still remained important to these young people and their families. This reflected the cultural importance of marriage in South Asian communities generally and impairment did not necessarily undermine this. Parents still wanted to ensure that, where possible, their sons and daughters with impairments had similar opportunities to their other children. The only two people who lived alone, Gurudev and Jaswant, had been divorced. Usually, however, the idea of living independently of the family home was rarely considered by the young people. They often explained this in terms of cultural expectations, although mentioning the limitations imposed by their impairment as well. Impairment or disability did indeed seem to affect the marriage negotiations, as differences emerged between the expectations of the young person and their brothers and sisters. As part of this, young people often felt they had to accept second best because of their impairment and believed the others in the family were more likely to find more suitable partners. Twenty-six-year-old Hardeep said that her sister had got the better husband:

"Compared to my husband, he's (her sister's husband) much cleverer, he speaks English and everything, he's more westernised. Yes I think I could have done better. I think the only reason I ended up with my husband is because of my disability. I ended up with him because of my leg. I know I could've done better."

Eight young people had married after becoming impaired. (The other three were married before the impairment.) In all but one case, their marriage partners came from India or Pakistan. Both parents and young people felt that it was easier to bring marriage partners from overseas rather than try to find marriage partners in the UK. Those who were considering marriage also said this. By comparison, their sisters and brothers seemed more likely to marry someone from the UK. There were various reasons given for seeking overseas marriage partners and most of the partners did seem to have been aware of the young person's impairment. Partners from overseas were seen as having lower expectations and so being more willing to come to the UK and look after someone. This is perhaps ironic given that some of the young people also felt that South Asian cultures were too 'backward looking', especially about disability. Young people and their parents also remarked that by considering marriage partners from South Asia they were offering their prospective partners the chance of settling in the UK. This, however, could have its disadvantages. Several young people and their parents were concerned that prospective partners were using marriage as an excuse to enter the UK and had no intention of trying to make the marriage work. Several young women, for instance, could tell of cases which confirmed their fears about this happening.

Being a woman also affected how the parents and young people felt about finding a suitable marriage partner. In some ways, women were seen to face greater difficulties because of cultural ideas about housework. Impairment was seen as affecting domestic work. This is why Fatima, aged 28 years, said that Asian women with impairments had a harder life than men:

"I don't know ... especially in our culture. Because you know, you have all these arranged marriages and it's like the guy comes to see you and obviously, like an Asian guy, he always expects a lot from his wife – he expects her to do the cooking, the cleaning and stuff like that and you've got someone with arthritis, you can't really, can you?"

Twenty-two-year-old Jamila similarly does not think she would be able to cope with married life, as she could not look after her husband properly.

The parents' part in arranging marriages was valued by their sons and daughters, as were ideas of family obligations. Nasira felt lucky to be married:

"I mean a lot of people wouldn't have given me a marriage partner but because it was my dad's brother's son he therefore agreed to marry me and I've been married for a long time now, but I know that a lot of girls wouldn't get married because nobody would give them a man to marry."

Finding marriage partners seemed to be different for women and men. Men were not only more likely to be married than women; they were also more likely to be engaged in the negotiations about marriage. Men, however, did face problems in fulfilling their role as 'breadwinners' and often felt that they were a 'burden' on their wives. Thirty-year-old Gurucharan, who became disabled because of a road accident, felt he was failing as a father and a husband:

"When you get disabled, it's not just that it affects you. You've got a family; you can't give them attention, like you're supposed to."

Gurucharan specifically felt he had become a 'burden' on his wife: "She's always mainly stressed out. She's got no time for herself".

Do these concerns about finding suitable marriage partners suggest that families give young people with impairments greater choice when considering potential marriage partners? Or is the way of negotiating the marriage – and all the expectations involved – the same for the young people and their sisters and brothers? All of them, it seemed, would take some part in marriage negotiations. Whatever changes impairment acceptability brings to this process, arrangements remained the same for all the family members. Most young people accepted this as a part of accepting their family's culture. Only three of the young disabled people considered marrying 'outside' their culture. Interestingly, all three of these had a strong sense of identity as a disabled person. They emphasised the importance of marrying someone who could 'cope' with their

disability; a feeling shared by one of the parents. Jagjeet's mother, for example, was concerned to ensure her daughter married a husband who would look after her:

"I would never arrange [a marriage] for her, because I, then that would be unfair because we could find her somebody but we do not know if he will care for her. So it's best she found somebody herself. I mean he does not have to be Indian. I won't mind as long as I knew genuinely in his heart that he would really look after her."

Summary

This chapter explored how young people saw the family and the prospect of marriage:

- Disability and impairment may be interpreted within the family in negative terms.
- This means there is often tension within families on this topic.
- It does not stop the young people from valuing the good relationships which they share with their families.
- Finding a partner, however, was part of life for the young people which they had to negotiate just as their brothers and sisters did. They were aware, however, that they would have more difficulty than their siblings in finding a marriage partner because of their impairment.

4

Disabling barriers and racism at work and at home

"I'll get angry, right, if they put me in cotton wool or something like that, if they watch me every minute."

The way young people saw the social effects of disability showed there was more to their lives than having an impairment. For example, they also experienced racism.

Young people had their own ideas about the lives they wanted to lead. Part of this was taking on other people's attitudes to disability. This included having to deal with the way in which their own parents treated them. Sometimes they felt that their parents had very negative views of disability, which reflected those of wider society. However, the young people, coped well with their parents views – it was a constantly changing process but they seemed able to recognise the support, care and love they received as well as the sometimes low expectations held about their abilities.

Sometimes young people shared their parents' negative views of disability. They often accepted their parents' ideas about their being at risk and tended to see impairment as a personal tragedy. These feelings seemed stronger among those who had become impaired as a result of illness or an accident. Thirty-year-old Gurucharan had severe physical impairments following a car accident:

"Like I say, my world's turned upside down. It's just a 100% different. I never envisaged life like this. All I can say is everything changed for me.... A lot of people say that I'm not the same person as before."

His own view was reinforced by those around him.

Young people often had to confront those barriers outside as well as within their family. Tahir, aged 19, was generally pleased with how his family treated him: "They just treat me as normal and stuff like that", although he felt that his family was "just a bit ashamed of themselves" for having a disabled child. This in turn makes him feel ashamed. Nineteen-year-old Shakeel felt different from his brother and sister: "You think you've let everyone down, that you're odd". Many young people felt isolated and undervalued within the family. Some, for instance, complained that despite the love shown by their families there was often little understanding of what they had to go through. Shakeel described his family as supportive but added:

"No one can understand you, even your own mother can't even understand how you feel, only you can, you know, how you feel. She obviously will hurt the most but she can never understand, no one can understand how you feel."

Many young people felt that their parents' poor view of disability drained away their own confidence. Nineteen-year-old Nargis said, "My family thinks I am useless; they're always putting my confidence down. That's why I'm a bit unconfident."

The disabled young people compared their experience with those of their brothers and sisters and felt that their parents treated the others more favourably. They commented that their parents gave the non-disabled children greater freedom (although, as we saw, brothers and sisters disagreed, often resenting the time that their parents spent with the disabled brother or sister). For the young person, there were also times when they felt that disability changed the usual age- and gender-related expectations; the roles which they would usually have taken were passed on to the other brothers and sisters. Young people resented such 'lack of respect', a term used repeatedly to describe their treatment by both their own family and other people. Some brothers and sisters, however, were sensitive to this. The younger brother of twenty-three-year-old Gurudyal said that he sometimes swapped roles with his brother: "Sometimes I am the younger, sometimes I am the older". He added that he was aware of how Gurudyal was prevented from assuming certain roles in the family because of his impairment – even with good intentions on the part of the rest of the family:

"I'm not thinking about marriage. Like in my family, the eldest gets married first. And I'm still trapped in that kind of, you know, thing, that the oldest gets married first. And, you know, I don't really want to get married first and that's going to be a bit of a problem. Because if I get married he's going to think, 'Oh I'm not married now' and he's going to say, he is going to start thinking."

The young people with impairments mentioned other worries about not being able to carry out family responsibilities, which made them feel useless. Some young people, for example, felt that they could not live up to what was expected of being a wife or husband. Several young women also felt they could not help their mothers with domestic work. Men worried about their role as 'breadwinners'. Some of the older respondents were worried about not being able to support their parents as they grew older. Waheed, aged 27 years, remarked:

"If I were an able-bodied person, when you get older, earning quite a lot of money, I would be able to look after them.... I sometimes do feel just a bit sad, but you know like I would not be able to look after them, you know, like I would have done if I had been an able-bodied person. Our culture is that the boy looks after his parents and his wife obviously."

Young people particularly disliked being dependent on other members of the family. They felt that this was 'not right', especially as they grew older. To this extent, young people directly compared their experience of 'growing up' with that of their brothers and sisters. They sometimes felt left out within the family as well as outside it in their social life.

'Overprotection'

Feeling overprotected caused tension between young people and their parents, reflecting some of the earlier difficulties mentioned. This went on throughout the young person's life. They saw their parents as feeling the need to protect them from the effects (as they saw them) of impairment and worrying about problems they might face while 'growing up'. Their parents often talked of the young person's well-being in terms of reducing risk. They recognised that they were overprotective sometimes but believed that they had no alternative. Several parents regretted not having given their children scope to develop their skills, especially as they got older and they saw the value of independence. Jagjeet's mother voiced a common dilemma faced by parents. She had raised all her children to be relatively independent, but she had failed to do this with her disabled daughter:

"I made a big mistake by doing everything for her, so now, it's not her fault, it's all my fault that I've made it too easy for her."

Generally the young people themselves felt that their parents were overprotective, especially when they compared their experiences to those of their brothers and sisters. Young people often saw their parents as overreacting to the difficulties they faced and, as they grew up with their own ideas, they questioned their parents' views of what was in their best interests. Other people of their age regarded South Asian parents' concerns as restrictive; the young people we interviewed felt it set them apart from others even more. They felt that they were being treated as children and they complained that their parents sometimes only saw their impairment and not just them as young adults. Nineteen-year-old Shakeel remarked: "I wish she [her mother] would like back off or something, you know give me more space". Twenty-six-year-old Hardeep Kaur described a similar problem. She said that her family was supportive, although they sometimes irritated her by worrying too much:

"I'll get angry, right, if they put me in cotton wool or something like that, if they watch me every minute."

They describe feeling that parents laid down restrictions rather than discussing them, which made it more difficult for the young person to accept. Challenging this sense of overprotection was not easy and the young people often felt guilty about upsetting their parents. Twenty-eight-year-old Fatima, for instance, said she did not know what she would do without her family, but added that this sometimes created problems:

"Sometimes it's good, you know, you get all the attention and you get everything done for you and then at other times, you wish you know, they wouldn't go on about it."

She was aware of being dependent at the same time as wanting to be independent.

Overprotection can be a common feature of any parent and child relationship. It may also be part of a parent's reaction to their child's growing sense of independence as well as a response to their son's or daughter's impairment. The parents' disabilist responses may be coming from the attitudes and ideas about disability which they see all around them. Comparing the accounts of the young people and their brothers and sisters confirmed that they did feel that they were treated differently. Waheed, aged 27, was aware that his parents treated him differently from his sister. This, however, may have been partly because he was an only son:

"I think if I had another brother, then they might not treat me like they do now. Part of it is because I'm disabled, but the other part is because I am the only one [son]."

Twenty-two-year-old Jamila said her parents were protective but she did not relate it to disability:

"I'm the youngest in the family so it's like, you know I'm their little baby, you know and they protect me too much."

Several young people with impairment felt that their parents were responding quite naturally to the risks associated with 'growing up' and that their parents had similar concerns for their other children. Being male or female as much as impairment also seemed to affect their response

to their children's independence. Parents were more protective of their daughters than their sons showing that impairment was only one important part of what is considered usual for someone of their own age, gender and social class.

The experience of twenty-eight-year-old Gurupal showed how complicated transition can be for young people. Like many young people he was 'growing up' disabled, with a sense of family religion and ethnicity, but in a Western culture and religion. Gurupal had to argue for greater independence:

"I think my disability is restricting, because they [parents] are more protective of what I do."

He specifically described his parents as too controlling:

"They seem very reluctant to let me have my freedom and sort of let me go in that respect. And I just want them to be more understanding and allow me to be my own person really."

He added, however, that his brother had also had problems about being independent. Gurupal felt his parents had different expectations of him than his brothers and sisters:

"I mean I love my family because they've been there and done everything for me, but their philosophies differ so much from what I think and I feel. I mean growing up in this country, I've learnt to accept their odd ways of doing things, but they were born and raised in a different culture, so their traditions and the way they do things different and I mean though they're trying to adapt and change to the way of living in the country. I think they find it hard whereas I'm born and raised here, so I haven't got any difficulty in adapting."

He had both insight and understanding of his parents' position.

Seeing disability within this broader context is also important in understanding how young people maintain a positive view of themselves. They seemed to see disability and the family as part of a whole picture of relationships. Nineteen-year-old Shakeel was aware of how much his family did for him, but at the same time he pointed out that they argued just like any other family:

"I don't know if I would be able to cope without my family. I need my family; I think definitely but yeah we fall out, you know, family things."

This way of looking at things also enabled the young people to play their part in the family, rather then just being a person with an impairment. It helped young people gain status by living up to the expectations associated with their role as a family member. There were many examples of them doing this. Young people in this study, for instance, were proud to support their parents and offer advice to other family members in the same way that Bignall and Butt (2000) found that driving a car was a useful role for young disabled people within their families.

Young people's views on disability

The negative family attitudes which the young people found disabling were also experienced outside the home. Thirty-year-old Gurucharan remarked:

"All I get from people is that they pity me type of thing, you know when they give you sympathy."

These attitudes annoyed him and showed how they made the young people feel devalued. Twenty-seven-year-old Waheed's account was typical:

"I mean I am not an able-bodied person but I don't feel bad about that. You know I feel that they [other people] treat you, they make your life just a little bit harder than actually what it is."

Robina, aged 27, agreed:

"The worst aspect is that people do not understand what makes your life difficult, but it's their kind of ignorance that annoys you sometimes and it gets you upset."

The young people with impairment felt that they missed opportunities and often compared

themselves to their brothers and sisters. Their ideas about getting married as mentioned earlier showed this. Education and work were another source of worry, particularly as they grew older. Feeling isolated was generally a problem for the young people we interviewed. Making friends was seen as part of being young and they identified with the popular images of fashion, film and TV and music. These symbols of youth culture as well as the mundane realities of school, work and home life were all important as a background to 'growing up'. Friends and outside contacts helped them to feel good about themselves. They wanted to meet other young people generally, not just young people with impairments. Disability, however, could limit the opportunities for such meetings and added to the young people's sense of being alone. This was in contrast to the experience of their non-disabled brothers and sisters, who, by and large, had wider and more frequent social contacts. Jagjeet contrasted her experience with that of her able-bodied brother:

"He can go where he wants because he ain't got no problem. I have to think of steps and stuff like, and toilet, but he doesn't have to worry about it because he is alright and he can take himself. I can't take myself. That really annoys me."

Eleven of the young people could describe few or no friendships beyond family life. In contrast, their brothers and sisters seemed to have no such problems in having a social life. Only two young people, Nargis (19 years old) and Shehnaz (29 years old), had the sort of social groups that they might have expected at their own age. Nineteen-year-old Shakeel was asked about what he did in his spare time. His response summed up the feelings of many other disabled young people: "Spare time? I think everyday is spare time for me". Shakeel commented that he could not keep up with his friends and therefore did not go out with them: "They got their own lives to live". Nasira found it difficult to make friends:

"I don't have any friends because I don't go anywhere, therefore I don't have any friends. They don't come around because I'm disabled, you see, they don't want to know me."

Twenty-seven-year-old Waseem felt angry and bitter about how his friends had treated him since he had become disabled:

"People used to know me, people used to visit me, they have all forgotten me. They all forget me."

Many of the young people and their families made a distinction between 'white' people's attitudes to disability and those of South Asian communities. Gurudev's mother, for instance, said that her son used to have more friends:

"It's just that our people are more scared of these things. If someone is disabled or something, our people are scared of them, rather than going up to talk to them and things like that. Our people are scared, white people just come and talk to him. It makes a difference."

Other parents and young people felt disablist attitudes had little to do with ethnic background. Surinder's mother, for instance, made no distinction between the white or South Asian community. She found them both to be equally dismissive and hostile to her family.

Dealing with discrimination

These examples of discrimination showed how the young people with impairment explained other people's behaviour in terms of the barriers which disabled them. Few young people discussed disability in a directly political way, however. Instead, they had a general view that they were missing out on opportunities, not just because of the practical limitations of impairment but also because of the insensitive attitudes of others which they felt held them back from doing what they wanted.

Some young people did see disability in a positive way, however, offering pride and resistance with which to fight against such negative views of disability. Twenty-eight-year-old Gurupal reflected on this discrimination:

"There's a lot of talented disabled people, who have got the ability to work and I think it's important that we're given the opportunity to showcase our abilities.... I don't think of myself as disabled. It's

society who's disabled by not enabling me to do this stuff. The most difficulty I experienced is through not being able to access buildings properly, not being able to get where I want to go because the facilities are not there to cater for me, so that's where I experience more discrimination really."

Twenty-two-year-old Jamila commented on the importance of how she saw herself: "I don't think negatively about myself. I think positive about myself". Contact with disabled people, as well as exposure to disability politics, helped support such views. Jagjeet explained:

"I find it easier to talk to [disabled people], because they are in a wheelchair, they know what it's like, it's brilliant because I find I'm more confident there."

Three young people, Shehnaz, Jaswant and Gurudev, were involved in organising activities for other disabled young people. All three stressed how important it was to meet others who could understand 'what you are going through', especially since they felt that their own families, despite their love and care, could not offer such understanding. These meetings also helped the young people to find out how to get in touch with services and the best ways of using the resources available to them. Such contact with others had helped Gurudev make sense of disability. He said:

"Disability carries a whole series of meanings, like sort of cut off from choices, your life, you are pigeon-holed."

Not everyone had access to these networks. With a few exceptions, even those who attended a day centre, where they met other disabled people, did not describe any sense of solidarity about being together. If anything they distanced themselves, comparing their situation to others, sometimes grateful that their situation was better, sometimes depressed because they felt that they had more difficulties than other disabled people. Some young people, although being aware of the disadvantages they faced, did not describe these disadvantages and discrimination in a political way.

The families' emphasis on trying to get the best for the young person with an impairment did mean, however, that they had some sympathy with the social effects of disability. They did not always use words like 'social model of disability', but they were aware of how society's failure to accommodate difference restricted the opportunities available to their child and of how they were 'disabled' by the response of others. Shushma's sister remarked that her brother was neglected by society:

> "I don't think enough provisions are made to make their quality of life better. It is simply a lack of understanding, people not accommodating."

Tahir's mother thought that the disadvantages faced by her nineteen-year-old son were made worse by other people's attitudes. She began by saying how her son had little social life:

> "He gets upset that he is not like others. He said 'I've nothing to get up for'. He didn't want to be bothered. Why should he get up? 'I've nothing to live for'."

She was not surprised, however, by her son's response:

> "Because when he goes out, they call him spastic and I think it is the most horrible word, 'Oh look at the spastic in the chair'. When he goes out people keep staring at him. It hurts him very bad."

Racism and disability

Culture can offer a chance to belong and can be politically important. The sense of being different, of experiencing disability discrimination and racism influenced how the South Asian young people we talked to made sense of their lives. To a large extent this discrimination happened with or without impairment. Nineteen-year-old Robina was one of the many young people who had experienced racism:

> "You get called Paki and things. It's not much more than anybody else would get I think. A lot of Asian people suffer that. I mean everybody comes across that at one point or another."

Waheed (aged 27 years) reflected on his experience of school: "They would call you Paki and why don't you go back where you come from?" Parents too were aware of this discrimination.

Young people's views on work

Although access to work may be seen as a common expectation for young adults, only six of the young people were in full-time work. Their brothers and sisters were more likely to be working and also to have better opportunities. Young people frequently compared their own situation with that of the rest of their family and felt that disability was one of the main reasons for any difference. Twenty-two-year-old Azhar reflected on the problems of finding a job and suggested that people "don't want a disabled person working for [them]". Nineteen-year-old Shakeel was aware that his impairment would make it difficult for him to get a job: "The employed will think this guy should be in care or something. They think I will not fit in". They were also aware that racism played its part. Nineteen-year-old Sohail was pessimistic about future employment because he was both Asian and disabled: "My cousins, they can't get a job, so it would be harder for me". Thirty-year-old Gurubax agreed:

> "I think at the end of the day you will have problems with the colour of your skin. That's a big problem, that on top of my disability. It does not make things easier."

Those who did work outside the home described various problems such as unhelpful workmates, teasing and cruel comments. The experience of twenty-two-year-old Afzar, for example, described the discrimination he faced at work:

> "They say I should stay at home. I don't know what's going on in their heads. They probably are saying what's that guy doing working here, you know. I was working Friday and this guy came up to me and said, 'What are you doing working here? You should be claiming benefits' and that."

Young people also found it difficult to get on at work, often because of the negative way in which other people saw impairment. Twenty-eight-year-old Gurupal was a journalist, but wanted to do more presenting work:

"It was very frustrating because I knew I had the ability to do the job. I had the talent but it was just the fact that I was physically unable to do it that prevented me from pursuing it further. When you see a presenter on television, he's very well groomed and he's very good looking and he's perfect. When a person is on television and he's in a wheelchair, people will be put off by seeing a disabled person."

There was very little formal support to help young people to find work. Once they had left school, most young people felt that they were forgotten about. Some of them relied on their families for support and encouragement. Some families felt that there should be more help for the young people with impairment and criticised the other people's poor expectations of what they could do. Tahir's mother said:

"I hope that there's somebody out there that does listen to him and give him a chance to get on with it. All these disabled people, surely they don't want to sit home the rest of their life?"

Other families were less encouraging. They themselves had negative views about impairment so some of them had low expectations of their children. Jagjeet, for instance, wanted to work in an office and had clear ideas about it: "I want to find a job, to work in an office, to be a secretary". Her mother, however, remarked, "She will not be able to work for anybody. She won't be able to get around much".

Summary

Young people's views of themselves were affected by the discrimination they experienced, which stopped them doing what they wanted to do:

- South Asian young people experienced disability discrimination in a similar way to that described by white young people.
- These negative views of impairment affected how they saw themselves.
- Some young people were becoming aware of how these barriers were preventing them from doing the things that they wanted to.
- They experienced racism at work and in the outside world generally.
- They also felt discriminated against at home because of disability.
- Young people saw being impaired as only one part of their identity. Being young, male or female, a part of their culture and religion and part of their families were seen as just as important.

5

Using the services

"They [teachers] used to say, 'oh you can't talk properly' … but I used to think sod them!"

One of the key things young people mentioned was how they dealt with things as their needs changed. They had to deal with 'growing up' just as their brothers and sisters did. Leaving school and finding work was part of that transition, as was learning to deal with social and health services as a young adult.

Education

Education is difficult for some young people with impairments of all ethnicities. As well as formal education, school offers a chance to make friends and meet people and enjoy yourself while learning new skills. Young people with impairments may lose out academically as well as socially. The academic level of 'special' provision may be poor, and the experience of those interviewed in our study supported this view.

The young people with impairments in mainstream schools found it hard to be positive about themselves, saying that they felt left out and undervalued because of their disability. They also felt that teachers thought that they were inferior to others without impairments. Many complained of being 'written off' by teachers. Nasira remarked:

"They [teachers] weren't interested in your work. If they wanted you to study, it was up to you, not to them."

She contrasted this with the support given to others in the class, who were not disabled. Twenty-two-year-old Jamila similarly described how she had difficulty in convincing her teachers to let her take GCSE exams:

"I had to fight like, to get what I wanted. So it was quite a struggle. They [teachers] discouraged me: 'You'll have difficulties doing some things because of your disability'. I had to argue with them all the time: 'No, it won't put me off, because I'm determined to do this'."

Eventually with her parents' help, she was given a three months' trial by the school to see if she could cope with the work. This proved successful and she was allowed to complete her GCSE courses.

Often there were not many other children with impairments at mainstream schools so the young people were mixing largely with non-impaired children. This meant that they then had access to mainstream youth culture. Sometimes, however, this contact was negative in terms of disability. Many young people described how they were teased at school, and were left feeling hurt and angry. Twenty-seven-year-old Robina explained:

"It's hard for you to understand why you're different and it's your fault, but these kids picking on you as well to add to that pain for you makes it really unhappy for you sometimes."

Being isolated at school was a problem for many young people, as Waheed, aged 27 years, remarked:

"The able-bodied people don't treat me as normal. And making friends, that was very hard. I felt lonely sometimes."

This kind of experience affected how young people felt about themselves and they commented on how hard it was to be confident. Nineteen-year-old Nargis, who is now at university, doubted that she would do sufficiently well in her GCSEs and 'A' levels to gain university entrance. No one at the school encouraged her:

"I thought I was sort of intelligent sometimes, but I thought, you know, I won't be able to do it."

However, some young people decided that it was important to challenge such negative views about impairments and fought back! Shehnaz remarked: "I handled it, I can usually give as good as I get from anybody." Azhar described his defiance:

"They just used to say, 'oh you can't talk properly' and this and that and 'he's handicapped and disabled', but I used to think, 'sod them'."

For some of them, these problems made them want to go to schools where children with impairments were taught together. The experience of those young people we interviewed who did attend 'segregated' schools did not support this view, however. Their biggest worry was about academic standards. Nineteen-year-old Tahir said:

"It's not like a proper school. It was just for the handicapped. It was a load of rubbish to me. It was just like typing something into the computer like kid's type stuff."

Parents shared these concerns. Gurupal's mother felt her son achieved little at a 'special' school, and she insisted that he was moved to a mainstream school:

"My idea was always to put him into a normal school because he was intelligent you know, he has got nothing wrong with his mind, it's just he's physically disabled, not mentally, so it was good when he did go to mainstream."

Gurupal agreed with his mother's assessment of his 'special' school and felt that no one took any interest in his education: "I wasn't treated like a human being in that school. I didn't feel that I was being treated properly". Like some of the other young people, however, academic achievement was not his only concern. He felt 'special' schools did not provide him with the skills to survive well outside school:

"If I would have been in a special school all my life I wouldn't have known how to interact and socialise with people who are able-bodied."

Some young people commented on the stigma of 'special' education. Twenty-eight-year-old Fatima said:

"I used to say, what am I doing in this school? I'm perfectly all right. I've got nothing wrong with me. I shouldn't be in this school."

Those who went to mainstream schools had a better academic record, with two young people going on to degree level education. Those who went to 'special' schools, on the other hand, were more likely to leave school with no formal qualifications. Nonetheless, nearly all the young people we interviewed had fewer qualifications than their brothers and sisters. Most left school to go to colleges of further education where they did basic courses such as information technology and life skills. Their brothers and sisters had more options open to them. The young people also saw these courses as having no real purpose, except to keep them occupied. Twenty-five-year-old Munir remarked: "It doesn't really matter ... it's just to get me out of the house and do something". This was a common view among those attending courses. Their parents agreed. Munir's mother, when asked about her son's course, said, "It passes the time". Young people often remarked on the stigma attached to such courses. Twenty-year-old Waheed completed a one-year life course at the college:

"[which showed] you how to wash your clothes, how to cross the road. I was so ashamed I couldn't tell my cousin what course I was doing, because it was a low course, but it was a course for mental people, and I wasn't mental."

Health and social services

Young people found it difficult to obtain the appropriate health and social services. Many commented on the problems of finding out about the support that was available to them. Twenty-seven-year-old Robina remarked: "I think information isn't readily available to you. I mean you have to go and search for it". Their parents also described similar problems. Moeen's mother did not know who to turn to for advice or help: "We don't even know what to do". Once they had discovered that help was available, young people often found it difficult to get hold of that support. They felt health and social care workers did not take their concerns seriously and sometimes made it difficult for them to get what they wanted. Several young people emphasised the importance of being demanding and not giving up in that situation. Twenty-two-year-old Azhar said:

"I've got to ask for it, it's part of life. You've got to ask, they don't come running to you do they?"

More generally, young people felt that workers did not listen to them and did not understand what they were going through. They felt that the services were insensitive and unsuitable. Many young people, therefore, had little confidence in welfare provision. Twenty-two-year-old Jamila went to a social worker to discuss the options available to her:

"I just wanted some information, you know, I was just deciding whether to move out and have my own place and he was like really putting me off, you know, saying, well, that's how I feel at the time, like he was saying, you know, it's really hard work, you have to, you've got your own place, you know, you've got the bills, you've got this and you've got that, you know, then you become lonely and stuff."

Their families also shared these concerns. Gurudyal's brother remarked that he felt that social services had lost interest in them because the family did not want to let Gurudyal go to live in an institution. Mushtaq's sister was especially critical of social workers:

"I mean social workers, they're just bloody stupid. No one gives a damn. The social workers are meant to be looking after him. But I don't think they do a good job."

There was a lack of trust between young people, their families and the service workers. Tahir's mother felt that the services constantly ignored her child's needs, despite requests for help. She said, "I don't trust them any more". The young people and their families often commented that having their needs recognised and acted on was a constant struggle. According to Rabia's mother, "When we request things, that is when things take forever". Nasira remarked: "The equipment that we use, we have to fight for it. We have to fight for everything".

Parents' views on welfare services

Parents, as we have seen, share their children's frustrations about service support, often acting as gatekeepers between their child and the services. As the child gets older, this role usually becomes less important. It may be different for young people with impairments. Parents were likely to be involved with services for far longer than they might have expected to for children without impairments. The young people themselves sometimes found this helpful and recognised that their parents were important allies in obtaining services. At the same time, young people were aware that service providers often let their parents speak for them. This left them feeling excluded. Several young people, for instance, mentioned that questions were directed at their parents when they felt that they should have been asked directly.

As well as being a proxy for their child, parents sometimes wanted professional help for themselves to meet their own and their children's needs appropriately. They often did not distinguish between this support for themselves and that for their child. This seems a common response among the families where a young person has an impairment. It can sometimes make the young person feel left out. Parents felt they got little support from the services, especially in coming to terms with their child's impairment (right from the time of diagnosis). The 'sense of loss' which they described seemed to be partly based on their contact with services where impairment was often presented to them as being a 'personal tragedy'. This meant that parents sometimes found it difficult to deal with impairment, feeling that their child was more at risk than others, would be in permanent need of support and have a restricted quality of life. Often these assumptions meant that they underestimated what their son or daughter could achieve.

The parents' relationships with services also reflected ambivalence. Some, for instance, were reluctant to accept support. Moeen's mother said:

> "I know there are carers that are available, but I want to look after Moeen myself. As far as I am concerned, as long as God gives me the energy to look after my son, I will. I don't want anybody else coming here and looking after my son."

Gurucharan's mother remarked:

> "He might think low of himself by saying that other people have to come and help. We therefore feel it is important that he knows we care."

Such comments might also reflect the parents' low expectations of the support available to them (as well as indicating how they felt about their own roles and responsibilities).

Appropriate services for minority ethnic groups

Many of these problems are typical of the contact between services and young people with impairments and their families – of any ethnic group. Insensitivity in welfare provision does, however, make the problems faced by South Asian young people and their families worse than disabled young people in general. The young people we interviewed faced some of the usual problems common to many minority ethnic groups in their dealings with the welfare state. Young people and their families could provide many examples where the communication with social workers, health professionals and the Benefit Agency hampered access to support. Young people and their parents also noticed crude stereotypes and myths being used by services. Impairment, for example, was often blamed by professionals on first-cousin marriage, as though the young person's impairment was only due to South Asian cultural practices. This made them feel blamed. More generally, young people and their families felt held back by their own limited access to the welfare state as well as by the service providers' failure to take account of all users' needs regardless of their ethnicity, background or of the language that they used.

Some young people and their parents also mentioned racism as a problem. Nasira, for example, was getting frustrated at trying to get social service support: "English people would have just got it, just like that". Nasira complained about the lack of facilities for South Asian people in particular:

> "There isn't anything there for us in terms of Asian people. Services aren't catered for us. English people know what they can get because they know what's available, but for Asian people its different, our needs are different."

When she challenged her local social services department she felt that they only stressed the problem of resources. Nasira was unhappy with this response:

> "They say they can't do anything for Asian people because they haven't got the money, but they do have the money because they have services for white people. Why don't they have them for Asian people?"

Both young people and their families believed that the services needed to understand and react to cultural differences. Their poor view of the services meant that they wanted better access to those services as well as to different kinds of support which recognised ethnic, cultural and religious differences.

Summary

In education, health and social services, young people and their families experienced:

- Racist and disabilist barriers to having their needs recognised and responded to by the welfare services.
- Limited opportunities because of the inability of services to recognise and deal with their needs.
- The need to be assertive about getting needs met.

6

Implications for policy, practice and research

The views of South Asian young people with impairments (together with those of their families) raised a number of important issues. Because little is known about what they think as opposed to what white people in the same situation think, the services may not always reflect what they want.

It is clear that services do fail to provide for them in the way that they want because providers do not know enough about their needs. Services may be based on stereotypes and myths about how South Asian people behave generally, for example, having lots of support from extended families. Another element that the services may focus on is the idea of independence which may be interpreted quite differently by South Asian people. An emphasis on leaving home, for instance, may not be the only way in which independence is defined. There are several ways in which disability and impairment are affected by age, gender and ethnicity, as well as religion and economics. How these young people saw the world did take account of all the other influences in their lives. They had clear ideas about what they wanted and they were quite used to compromising between their families' ideas and their own as well as with those of wider society.

Negative views of impairment and disability did affect them and make them feel discriminated against. Sometimes these views came from their parents, extended families or from their communities. Some of them had learnt to deal with this disability discrimination in the same kind of ways in which they dealt with racial discrimination. They also found that they could take their families' culture and religion and use it as a part of their own view of the world. Some found disability politics useful, others found

family support an effective way of dealing with the world. They deal with disability, discrimination, racism and living in different cultures and religions at the same time as all the other aspects of growing up.

Learning about ethnicity, culture and religion

Ethnicity was not neutral and it included language, culture, religion and nationality, as well as a shared history. It was important to look at how the young people saw ethnicity. Contact with their parents' country of origin was a symbol of ethnic identity and, as such, links were important for nearly all the parents we interviewed, as was the use of their first language. Young people, however, were less enthusiastic about their parents' countries of origin and language. They shared similar views to their brothers and sisters and to other South Asian young people living in Britain. They and their brothers and sisters identified with being 'British' more than with being 'Pakistani' or 'Indian'. Their sense of being British was often based on being born and living in Britain. There was also a view that the attitudes and values held by the South Asian community living in Britain were less restrictive than those in their parents' homeland. Young people with impairments, particularly, found identification with Britishness as being even more important because they felt that they received more 'respect' within 'British' than 'Asian' situations and had access to better support. Learning their parental language was more acceptable and many spoke more than one language, but some had been 'let off' learning on the grounds of disability.

Young people's responses to their own or their parents' country of origin often saddened their parents. Parents' attitudes to their homeland also varied. If parents had little interest it was also likely that both the young person and their brothers and sisters had weak ties with their parents' country of birth and only limited understanding of their parents' language. The young person's impairment played only a small part in this. Access to religious teaching was a particular problem for young people – there was little disabled access provided by formal religious institutions and attitudes of religious teachers were often disablist.

How their families responded to religion was also important. Religion was an important aspect of identity for South Asian young people living in Britain. The young people we interviewed sometimes said that their disability interfered with their sense of religion. They had poor access to the wider community networks that might have helped to develop religious and cultural connections. This problem seemed to be about the more formal practice of religion. None of the young people we interviewed was completely removed from their parents' ethnic, religious and cultural traditions. Most had a working knowledge of religion and culture and did identify with their family's religion. In many ways, young people had a similar awareness of religious and cultural values to their brothers and sisters, although many had only limited access to formal religious teaching. Where it was limited it was likely that it was shared by the rest of the younger generation of the family.

Young people with impairment and their sisters and brothers understood how to work through these conflicts. Those conflicts that did arise with their parents were often a result of different understandings of cultural values rather than a lack of knowledge. Young Muslim women, for example, could question their parents' restrictions on Western dress, while still recognising the importance of modesty. This showed the success of the families' ability to pass on ethnic, religious and cultural values. It also reduced the impact of the child's impairment as a separate issue on learning about family, religion and culture.

Relationships and disability

South Asian parents faced similar difficulties of providing practical, social and financial support to those described in the general literature on young people's impairment and chronic illness. They also sometimes held negative views of the effect of disability on their family, partly because of how it was presented to them initially by professionals.

Young people with impairments shared some of their parents' and wider family's negative views, but not all. This led to a tension in the stories young people and their families told. The young people accepted that they might be at risk, but at the same time they wanted to lead valuable lives. Some young people felt that their parents' view of disability undermined their own confidence. They felt left out in some situations but they also felt a part of the loving and caring families, which often helped compensate for such negative views and experiences.

The young people saw parents as allies trying to secure the best opportunities for them. All of them were aware of how society did not accommodate impairment and difference and restricted the opportunities available to these young people – they all saw clearly the social effects of disability.

Overprotection caused tension between young people and their parents. The young people often interpreted their parents' actions as an overreaction to the difficulties they faced. Gender was significant here, as young women within South Asian communities felt that they were seen as having more easily damaged reputations. Moral protection of young women was part of a general cultural picture, and such protection did restrict the social lives of young women more than young men with impairments.

All the young people had to engage with their parents over rules and negotiations. Comparing the accounts of the young people with impairment with those of their brothers and sisters confirmed this. Young people with impairments had to 'grow up' in the same way as their peers. Seeing impairment in this broader light helped young people to have a good view of themselves. They recognised that impairment was only one part of their lives. That is why young people gained a lot by fulfilling expectations of their roles as family members – giving advice or in helping other people.

Young people and their families often criticised the extended family for having a negative view of disability. They sometimes felt socially isolated and ostracised, and wished that their extended families were more accommodating and understanding.

The social meaning of disability

The negative views of impairment that young people found in the family were similar to those outside. They felt that people underestimated them. Young people also felt that, compared to their brothers and sisters, they were denied opportunities socially. They faced discrimination in education and at work, and were often denied the opportunities available to their brothers and sisters. They also found it more difficult to find a marriage partner and to leave the family home if they wanted to, as well as fulfil the family obligations which they saw as usual for someone of their age and gender. Isolation was a particular problem for young people and this also contrasted with the experience of their brothers and sisters who did not have impairments.

Discrimination accounted for why some young people, like their parents, were drawn towards explanations of disability. Few young people discussed this in a political way, though they did describe barriers. As with their parents, young people's stories reflected both social and medical explanations of disability. A few young people had taken a more positive political view of disability and drew strength from this.

This positive identity as a disabled person had advantages for them but they still felt that some of it may have been based on Eurocentric ideas. Independence, for example, may not have had the same meaning among different ethnic groups. Policy and practice needs to take account of this difference in outlook.

Just as Bignall and Butt (2000) found in their study of young black people with impairment, independence had many different meanings. Sometimes it was about living on your own or about making choices about how you spent your time or which colour your room was painted. At other times it was about taking control. There

was a clear expectation that young people growing up become more self-reliant and less dependent on others, and this may be affected by impairment and disability. It is still closely linked to family relationships where give and take and depending on each other is important.

South Asian young people wished to be part of their ethnicity, culture and religion and this influenced their experience of disability. Discussion has tended to concentrate on 'cultural conflict' between South Asian young people and their parents, but in our study we saw quite a successful way of dealing with cultures and religions among the young people with impairments.

Use of the services

As well as being part of identity, family culture and ethnicity can also have another political effect, that of being excluded by a powerful majority. A sense of difference, emphasised by racism and discrimination, remained an important influence on how these South Asian young people saw their lives. Racism, for example, was a feature of the young person's relationship to services. Young people and their families, for example, sometimes found services unable to respond to their needs or were treated according to racial myths and stereotypes that denied them the support that they needed. The young person's disability added to this discrimination and affected how much they would control their lives. Some of this disablist discrimination was shared with their 'white' disabled peers. Generally, however, disablist barriers and racism meant that South Asian young people with impairments – and their families – had difficulties in getting the right kind of services from the welfare state.

Social views of disability

Disabling barriers were a powerful influence on how these young South Asian people saw themselves. Young people had to deal with disablist views, both from within their family and outside, suggesting that disabled people have much in common irrespective of ethnic origin. Explanations of these barriers, however, have often been based on white people's experiences.

Our findings suggest that impairment can only be made sense of within the whole picture of someone's life. Most young people saw themselves as defined by other things as well as impairment. Both racism and disablism affected how young people saw themselves, but so did their age and gender.

We talked mainly with Pakistani Muslims and some Sikhs. They reported similar experiences and perspectives, which may suggest that the findings are likely to apply to South Asian groups more generally.

Policy and practice need to reflect this diversity and not assume that Western ideas about disability and independence have the same meaning for South Asian young people and their families. In particular, services need to become more sensitive to the cultural and religious values held by young people and their families and to recognise how these interact with the experience of disability. Doing this will help to make sure that services are better informed about what minority ethnic people with impairments and their families themselves want, rather than basing it on various disablist and racist stereotypes.

Bibliography

Afshar, H. and Maynard, M. (1994) *The dynamics of 'race' and gender*, London: Taylor and Francis.

Ahmad, W.I.U. (1996) 'Family obligations and social change in Asian families', in W.I.U. Ahmad and K. Atkin (eds) *'Race' and community care*, Buckingham: Open University Press.

Ahmad, W.I.U. (2000) *Ethnicity, disability and chronic illness*, Buckingham: Open University Press.

Ahmad, W.I.U. and Atkin, K. (1996) *'Race' and community care*, Buckingham: Open University Press.

Ahmad, W.I.U, Darr, A., Jones, L. and Nisar, G. (1998) *Deafness and ethnicity: Services, policy and politics*, Bristol/York: The Policy Press/ Joseph Rowntree Foundation.

Armstrong, F. and Barton, L (1999) *Disability, human rights and education*, Buckingham: Open University Press.

Atkin, K. and Rollings, J. (1996) 'Looking after their own? Family caregiving among Asian and Afro-Caribbean communities', in W.I.U. Ahmad and K. Atkin (eds) *'Race' and community care*, Buckingham: Open University Press, pp 73-86.

Barnes, C. Mercer, G. and Shakespeare, T. (1999) *Exploring disability: A sociological introduction*, Cambridge: Polity Press.

Beresford, B. (1994) *Expert opinions: A national survey of parents caring for a severely disabled child*, Bristol/York: The Policy Press/Joseph Rowntree Foundation.

Beresford, B., Sloper, P., Baldwin, S. and Newman, T. (1996) *What works in services for families with a disabled child?*, Barkingside: Barnardos.

Bignall, T. and Butt, J. (2000) *Between ambition and achievement: Young black disabled people's views and experiences of independence and independent living*, Bristol/York: The Policy Press/Joseph Rowntree Foundation.

Brannen, J., Dodd, K., Oakley, A. and Storey, P. (1994) *Young people, health and family life*, Buckingham: Open University Press.

Chamba, R., Hirst, M., Lawton, D., Ahmad, W. and Beresford, B. (1999) *Expert voices: A national survey of minority ethnic parents caring for a severely disabled child*, Bristol: The Policy Press.

Corker, M. and French, S. (1998) *Disability discourse*, Buckingham: Open University Press.

Drury, B. (1991) 'Sikh girls and the maintenance of ethnic culture', *New Community*, vol 17, no 3, pp 387-99.

Finch, J. and Mason, J. (1994) *Negotiating family responsibilities*, London: Routledge.

Finklestein, V. (1993) 'The commonality of disability', in J. Swain, V. Finklestein, S. French and M. Oliver (eds) *Disabling barriers – enabling environments*, London: Sage Publications, pp 126-32.

Hill, M. (1993) 'They're not our brothers: the disability movement and the black disability movement', in N. Begum, M. Hill, and A. Stevens (eds) *Reflections: Views of black disabled people on their lives and community care*, London: CCETSW, pp 68-80.

Hirst, M. and Baldwin, S. (1994) *Unequal opportunities: Growing up disabled*, London: HMSO.

Katbamna, S., Bhakta, P. And Parker, G. (2000) 'Perceptions of disability and care giving relationships among South Asian communities', in W.I.U. Ahmad (ed) *Ethnicity, disability and chronic illness*, Buckingham: Open University Press, pp 12-27.

Modood, T., Beishon, S. and Virdee, S. (1994) *Changing ethnic identities*, London: Policy Studies Institute.

Modood, T., Berthoud, R., Lakey, J., Nazroo, J., Smith, P., Virdee, S. and Beishon, S. (1997) *Ethnic minorities in Britain: Diversity and disadvantage*, London: Policy Studies Institute.

Morris, J. (1993) *Community care, independent living and disabled people*, Basingstoke: Macmillan.

Oliver, M. (1996) *Understanding disability: From theory to practice*, Basingstoke: Macmillan.

Priestley, M. (1999) *Disability, politics and community care*, London: Jessica Kingsley.

Roulstone, A. (1998) *Enabling technology: Disabled people, work and new technology*, Buckingham: Open University Press.

SSI (Social Services Inspectorate) (1998) *They look after their own, don't they?*, London: SSI.

SSI (2000) *Excellence not excuses: A jigsaw of services*, London: SSI.

Stuart, O (1996) 'Yes, we mean black disabled people too', in W.I.U. Ahmad and K. Atkin (eds) *'Race' and community care*, Buckingham: Open University Press, pp 89-104.

Appendix

More about the young people interviewed:

Age

1 aged 17-18
6 aged 19-20
5 aged 21-22
2 aged 23-24
2 aged 25-26
7 aged 27-28
6 aged 29-30

Status

Eight were at college, one at university and nine on training courses. Four others were working. Most lived at home with their parents. Eleven were married and two were divorced.

Families

14 parents (5 fathers, 9 mothers)
15 brothers and sisters (9 brothers, 6 sisters)

Interviews

Interviews in Punjabi and Urdu were translated into English. Two people refused to be tape-recorded so notes were taken.

We used qualitative methods to analyse the interviews onto a map or framework using the themes which came up. We compared them and looked at the different backgrounds to try and develop ideas from these which would be useful to inform the services.

As well as contacts through statutory and voluntary groups, community members were consulted to contact young South Asian people with impairments.